Restless Legs Syndrome Treatment

Learn What Causes Restless Legs, How to Deal with the Symptoms Naturally and Effectively, How to Relax and Finally Let Your Legs Rest

By Emma D. Jones

3

Table of Contents

Introduction

Also referred to as Willis-Ekbom disease, Restless Legs Syndrome (RLS) is a condition in which your legs feel uncomfortable sensations. These sensations can be in the form of tingly, creeping, and crawling feelings, which create an overwhelming desire to move the affected leg(s).

These very uncomfortable symptoms usually occur when the afflicted person is sitting, resting, or sleeping and are most evident at nighttime. These symptoms or feelings of discomfort along with an overwhelming urge for movement are caused due to RLS and are known as periodic limb movements of sleep or (PLMS). These movements can cause a lot of sleep issues for the afflicted person.

Primary RLS usually has no discernible cause whereas secondary RLS can occur because of pregnancy, nerve issues, chronic kidney failure or iron deficiency. While mild symptoms of RLS have little or no impact on the patient's lifestyle, moderate to severe symptoms can turn a person's life completely awry.

Lack of restful sleep caused by moderate to severe symptoms of RLS can be debilitating. Lack of sleep can result in lack of focus and concentration during daytime taking its toll on your social activities, and worse still, on your job. These problems will, in turn, lead to anxiety and stress. The longer you take to manage RLS, the more difficult your life will become. Moreover, if left unattended, symptoms of RLS can spread to other parts of your body like to your arms.

As RLS has a direct impact on your life, it makes sense to spend time, energy and other resources to treat the disease or, at least, keep the symptoms in check. There are various methods of treating RLS. The lack of a standard method is due to the fact that its causes are difficult to identify and are not really clear.

Some researchers are of the opinion that RLS is caused by the damaged working of the chemicals in the brain while others opine that it is caused due to the inefficient working of the circulatory system. Although the next chapter is dedicated to causes, symptoms and other theoretical aspects of Restless Legs Syndrome, the rest of the book is dedicated to homemade, natural and lifestyle remedies for this malady.

While medications for the disease should be taken only on the advice of a qualified medical practitioner, most of the suggestions and tips given in this book are natural and based on lifestyle modifications including the right kind of nutrition and exercises to follow. In addition, I have included a few relaxation techniques including yoga and meditation and the use of some essential oils and herbs with the potential to reduce symptoms and pain for the patient.

So, go on and read on to find out more about Restless Legs Syndrome and many natural remedies for it.

Chapter One:

Diagnosis, Causes, and Symptoms of Restless Legs Syndrome

While it is good to have remedies in place, it makes sense to spend a little time to understand the diagnoses, causes and symptoms of RLS to better understand the right method of treatment to take.

Diagnosis

At present, there are no medical tests to diagnose restless legs syndrome. Yet, medical practitioners conduct tests and counter-tests to rule out other conditions with similar symptoms. The diagnostic approach to RLS includes:

- Symptoms as reported by the patient
- Answers to questions regarding family history, use of medication
- Presence or absence of other conditions and their symptoms
- Problems associated with daytime sleepiness

Yes, it is rather tricky to correctly diagnose this medical condition. Moreover, even if you were to go by the symptoms (which are explained in the next subheading), all of the symptoms are not present at all times leading to even more confusion than before.

Another problem with the symptoms is the fact that it is almost impossible to replicate while you are visiting the doctor as most often, the symptoms are in their highest intensity during night time when the patient is sleeping (or rather trying to sleep).

Some people do have the symptoms of RLS even when they are resting during the day. Yet, it is less severe and not very obvious to others. These symptoms get worse as evening sets in and reach intensely severe levels at nighttime.

So, the doctor has to rely on the patient's description of the symptoms for diagnosing the condition rather than any imaging techniques and/or lab tests. Therefore, it is essential that, as a patient, you learn to self-diagnose the condition because you are the one who understands and feels the pain of the symptoms.

As the patient, you will be able to identify the characteristic symptoms earlier on and be sure enough to rule out other causes and then try some home remedies for the problem.

Symptoms

The following are the characteristic symptoms of restless legs syndrome:

- A clearly uncomfortable sensation in your legs along with an almost irresistible urge to move or flex your limbs
- A temporary feeling of relief from the uncomfortable sensations when you flex or move your legs
- The symptoms get aggravated during resting and sleeping times
- The symptoms gradually get worse as evening approaches
- It gets very difficult to fall asleep because of these symptoms waking you up often during nighttime sleep

The first four symptoms listed above are essential to be clinically diagnosed with restless legs syndrome. However, if the last symptom also exists, then you must take professional advice because the lack of restful sleep (or insomnia) increases the risk of depression, hypertension and other cardiovascular disorders.

These uneasy and uncomfortable sensations can be described as:

- A pulling or a creeping sensation
- An itchy feeling that you cannot scratch away
- A persistent dull ache in the legs, sometimes becoming painful
- A sense of restlessness resulting in pacing the room at nights, tossing and turning on the bed and rubbing of legs

In severe cases of RLS, the person will not feel any relief even with sufficient movement of the legs. Although the name of the disorder is restless legs syndrome, these symptoms can affect even other parts of the body including neck, hands and the entire body as well.

Many RLS-afflicted patients are also prone to another medical condition called PLMS or periodic limb movements in sleep, which can create a lot of sleep disturbances both for the patient and his or her partner. PLMS is characterized by jerking, involuntary, periodic and repetitive limb movements while sleeping, resting, or in severe cases, even when the patient is awake and is involved in some activity.

Some people with RLS may not feel sustained symptoms. It might come for a few days and there could be days or even months when they don't feel the symptoms. Then there could be remission of symptoms that come unannounced or without warning.

Causes / High-Risk Individuals

The following people are known to carry a high risk of being afflicted by RLS.

Gender – While RLS can affect people of both genders, women are generally more susceptible than men. Pregnancy enhances the risk. Of the women who got RLS during pregnancy, some could be completed cured of it while some women could get a long-term remission after delivery.

Age – RLS is known to be more prevalent among people who are older than 40 years rather than younger people. However, there are many cases of RLS among 20-somethings and even among children and teenagers.

Lifestyle – A sedentary lifestyle, consumption of alcohol and smoking are all known to increase the risk of RLS.

Food and Drugs – Caffeinated foods and medications for various physical and psychological disorders are known to increase the risk of RLS or enhance the intensity of the symptoms. Medications that have the potential to trigger RLS symptoms include antidepressants, sedatives, antihistamines and opioids.

Other medical problems – Diabetes, obesity, anemic disorders, Parkinson's disease and other nerve-related disorders could trigger RLS too

Genetics – Most of the people with RLS have a family history of the disorder. Genetic researchers and experts have found many genes that carry the risk of RLS. It has been seen that people with RLS invariably have others in their family who are also affected by it.

So, you can see that restless legs syndrome cannot really be diagnosed through tests or imagery techniques. A lot of the information has to come from the patient. It is imperative that if you suspect RLS as a problem, then you must be very sensitive to the characteristic symptoms mentioned above.

Effective treatments for RLS are not only elusive but also the failures of repeated attempts can frustrate even the most dedicated patient. In addition to medications, it is good to work with alternative therapeutics to result in optimum benefits for you. You can work with your physician and create a treatment regimen that combines the natural remedies with what your doctor prescribes for best results. From the next chapter onwards, this book is dedicated to giving various natural remedies through exercise, food, etc.

Chapter Two:

Exercises Remedies for RLS

There are multiple exercises that are known to relieve stress and pain associated with restless legs syndrome. Moderate to mild forms of exercises done regularly, preferably on a daily basis, is one of the most effective natural remedies for restless legs syndrome. These exercises are non-invasive and not very difficult to learn and master.

It is important to keep the intensity of exercises at a moderate level. There are many ex-marathoners who are frustrated about having to tone down the intensity of their workouts after being diagnosed with RLS. However, medical experts and professionals caution that this is the only way to reduce and ease the pains and agonies of RLS.

Effects of Exercising on RLS Patients

Exercises ease the pain of RLS symptoms in many ways and some of them are:

- Exercising triggers complex biochemical reactions in the body that increases blood flow to the muscles in the leg.
- Exercising triggers the release of endorphins or the feel-good hormones that facilitate stress reduction, which, in turn, promotes sleep.

- Exercising increases the production and release of dopamine which has a direct impact on reducing the effects of pain
- Regular exercise regimens help in weight management and reduction of belly fat both of which are connected to RLS

It is important that you check with your physician before starting off with any exercises to try managing RLS.

Tips for Exercising

Exercise thrice a week, at least – Combining aerobic exercises and resistance training for the lower body is an effective exercise regimen for controlling and managing RLS symptoms. Your exercise regimen should be for at least three times a week for optimum results. Experts recommend starting at 30-minute workouts and then slowly increasing the duration to about an hour over a period of six months.

Avoid exercising just before going to bed – Early morning is the most effective time for exercising. If you find it difficult to do it first thing in the morning, at least finish it by the afternoon. Exercising even 3-4 hours before your bedtime can trigger RLS symptoms making it difficult for you to fall asleep.

Avoid high intensity and high impact exercises – This means long-distance cycling, running, jogging, lifting heavy weights, kickboxing, spinning and all such workouts must be avoided. There are research studies, which prove that strenuous exercises can trigger RLS symptoms by inflaming and irritating leg tissues. High impact exercises are essentially those that require you to employ large muscles in your body to propel yourself into the air or lifting both your feet off the ground. Similarly, strenuous forms of yoga like the Ashtanga Yoga are to be avoided for RLS. Power hiking or power walking is also a no-no.

Indulge only in low-intensity and low-impact exercises – Moderate and gentle exercise regimens are critical for reducing RLS symptoms. Gentle stretching, walking, cycling, balancing exercises, gentle yoga postures, etc. are recommended. Low impact aerobics where one foot is always in touch with the ground is good too. Wear sturdy shoes to avoid excessive pressure and stress on the legs.

Train with caution – If your RLS symptoms are severe, you need to take extra caution during your training regimens. Avoid elliptical machines, treadmills, leg presses, etc. Instead train on those machines that work on your abdomen, arms and your shoulder muscles. Experts also advise using only one machine. Using multiple machines can also trigger RLS symptoms.

Gentle squats are good – Squats are good for RLS because they increase the flow of blood to the legs thereby reducing RLS symptoms. To do a squat, stand straight with your arms outstretched ensuring your back is straight too. Now, squat down until your thighs and the floor are parallel. Now, slowly get back to your standing position. Repeat not more than 2-3 times. Excessive repetition can also trigger RLS symptoms.

Swimming and water aerobics are great too – As swimming and water aerobics take the weight off your legs, they are excellent to reduce symptoms of RLS. Using a float to keep your legs above the floor of the pool will enhance the effectiveness of water aerobics.

Exercises and Stretches for RLS

Try some of the following exercises and stretches at home. Repeat them slowly and increase intensity and duration gradually over time for maximum benefit.

Seated Position Exercises

Heel-to-Toe Rock – Place your foot on the floor and first lift your heel. Then, replace your heel onto the ground and lift the toes. Alternate between the heels and toes and repeat five times.

Heel Push – Place your feet close to the chair and lift the heels of both the legs so high that only the balls of your feet are touching the ground. Now, bend slightly forward ensuring your back is straight and place both your hands on your right knee. Use the power and strength of your upper body to push the heel of the right leg to the floor. Raise the heel again and repeat the exercise for five rounds. Next, place your hands on the left leg and repeat the exercise

Knee-to-Chest – Place your left hand under your left thigh close to the knee. Gently and slowly, push the knee towards your chest and back. Repeat five times. Repeat for the other leg too. The next level could include ankle circles. Here's how you do it. Lift your knee in the same way and hold it in position. Now, circle the ankle 5 times in the clockwise and anticlockwise directions. Repeat for the other leg too. If you are suffering from osteoporosis, then this knee-to-chest exercise is better to be avoided.

Ankle Motion – Straighten one leg so that it is parallel to the ground. Then, point and flex the toes of the leg five times. Then, rock your ankle from side to side like you are waving goodbye with your feet. Repeat with the other leg too.

Ankle Rotation - Sit on a chair at the edge with both feet planted firmly on the ground. Lift your left foot about 3 inches off the floor and point your toes toward the floor. Using your toes like a pen, draw a circle toward your right while keeping the rest of the leg still. Draw about 10 circles and put your left foot gently on the floor. Now, repeat with your right foot too.

Standing Position Exercises

Soleus Stretch – Step back with one foot in such a way that the toes of this foot are along the heel of the other foot. Keeping your feet and heels firmly on the ground, go down vertically by bending your knee. Ensure your torso is erect. You will feel a stretch above the heel cord on the leg that is at the back. Hold this position for about 10 seconds. Revert back to the original standing position and repeat with the other leg.

Gastroc Stretch – Hold the back of a sturdy chair for support and stand straight. Take a big step back with your left foot. Now, bend the right knee while keeping the left knee straight. Keeping the toes of both the feet pointed in the forward direction, press down the heel of the left leg (which is at the back). You will feel a stretch in the calf muscle of the left leg. Hold this position for about 10 seconds. Then release it by lifting the heel off from the ground. Repeat the press and release posture five times. Then, come back to the standing position and repeat with the right leg.

Hamstring Stretch – Start the same way as you did for the gastroc stretch until you took that big step back with your left leg. Keep your left leg straight with your knees slightly bent for added support. Now, lift the toes of your right leg (which is forward) and bend a little at the hips keeping the heel touching the ground.

Now, pull the toes of the right leg forward as if you are trying to bring it close to your shin. At this point, you will feel the stretch at the thigh muscles of your right leg. Hold this position for 10 seconds. Now, get back to the original standing and repeat with the other leg.

Calf Stretch – Take a big step forward with your right leg and bend the right knee so that it is level with the ankle. Keep your left leg firmly pressed to the ground and the knees straight. You will feel the stretch of the calf muscles of the left leg. Hold it for 10 seconds and come back to the standing position. Now repeat for the right leg calf stretch.

Hip Stretch – Place a chair in front of you and place your back against the wall. Now, lift your right leg and place the foot flat on the chair that is in front of you. For this, you will have to bend your right knee. Now, making sure your backbone is straight, bend forward slightly at the hips. As you bend more, you will feel the top of the right thigh stretching. Hold for 10-20 seconds and get back to position. Now, repeat with the left thigh.

Other Exercises for RLS

These exercises can be done while in the seating or standing positions. Do what is comfortable for you.

Bounce - on your heels ensuring the movements are gentle and small. It is important to slowly try and get into a rhythm of bouncing on your heels. It will come with patient practice.

Shake – one leg gently by lifting it off the ground. Repeat for the other leg as well.

March – First, march on your toes only. Next, march on your heels only. Lastly, march on your entire feet.

Pat and Tap Your Legs – With open palms, pat and tap your legs in the upward and downward movements.

Walking – Walking sounds like a very simple thing to do and yet, if you speak to people, you will realize that this is one of the exercise elements that are left out of their regular regimen. A regular 30-minute walk every day can relieve RLS symptoms significantly.

Find a time that is convenient for you and make sure you do a good brisk walk without crossing over to the high-intensity, high-impact range. A short walk after your lunch if you cannot do it as soon as you get up is a great way to make sure you get your daily dose of walking.

Walking works your thigh and calf muscles, gets the blood flowing through your body, and gives you a fabulous cardio workout. Daily walking can improve your sleep patterns and reduce RLS symptoms to a large extent. So, take your daily walk without fail.

Some More Leg Stretches

Seated Calf Stretch – This exercise will be good to relieve cramps in the night, which are preventing you from sleeping. Sit on the bed and stretch out your left leg. Flex your left leg toward you. Wrap both your palms around your left foot and pull the toes toward you. Hold this position for about 10-20 counts. If you cannot reach your palms around your foot, use a scarf or a towel to pull the toes towards you. Go back to the original position and repeat for the right leg as well.

Find the best exercise routine that suits you and your lifestyle. While some people like to finish off their exercise regimen first thing in the morning, others would prefer to do it in the evening though you must ensure it is at least 5-6 hours before bedtime. You can choose the set of exercises, stretches, and mild-to-moderate cardio regimens that fit into your routine well.

Chapter Three:

Nutritional Remedies for RLS

Iron and Restless Legs Syndrome

More and more studies are revealing a connection between iron deficiency and RLS. Iron is one of the primary elements needed for hemoglobin synthesis. Hemoglobin is the red pigment in blood that is responsible for carrying oxygen to all parts of the body.

When iron levels are low, hemoglobin functioning and synthesis are compromised resulting in reduced oxygenation in tissues and cells. These actions take place even before the anemia resulting from iron deficiency actually sets in and can be measured.

Iron is also an important element for the production of dopamine, a chemical produced in the brain used for muscle and nerve co-ordination. Recent research studies have increasingly proven that there is a clear connection between RLS and abnormal functioning and production of dopamine. In fact, physicians prescribe drugs that enhance dopamine production for cases with severe RLS symptoms.

Your physician is sure to check your iron levels in your blood if you approach him or her for solutions for RLS. Instead of merely checking for hemoglobin levels, your physician will check for the level of ferritin in your blood. Ferritin is an iron-binding protein found in the blood.

Measuring the level of ferritin is a more sensitive method of correctly identifying the level of iron in your blood instead of checking for hemoglobin levels. If the reading for ferritin is on the lower side, your doctor will most likely ask you to consume foods with extra iron content or take supplements.

Foods Rich in Iron – Red meats, liver, dark green leafy vegetables like spinach, dry fruits, poultry, pork, seafood and beans are rich sources of iron. Increase the intake of foods cooked with these ingredients. Moreover, eating foods rich in Vitamin C enhances the ability of your body to absorb iron better. Foods rich in Vitamin C include melons, citrus fruits and broccoli.

Magnesium and Restless Legs Syndrome

Magnesium is a mineral needed by our bodies for the smooth functioning and regulation of several biochemical reactions. Magnesium is an essential element for proper nerve and muscular functions and for a healthy immune system. Low levels of magnesium could lead to problems associated with the conduction of nerve impulses, muscle cramps and muscle contractions.

There are research studies that prove the connection between low levels of magnesium and RLS. Magnesium is used as an alternative therapy for RLS, especially if it is suspected that its deficiency is a probable cause for the condition.

Many experts and researchers believe that magnesium in the body facilitates the easy relaxation of muscles. The reason for this is attributed to the calcium-blocking attributes of magnesium, which help in regulating nerves and muscles to relax countering the 'activation' function of calcium. When magnesium levels are low in the body, calcium is not able to be blocked resulting in overactive nerves and muscle contractions. Therefore, experts believe that if magnesium is a contributory factor to the RLS condition, then magnesium supplement or food rich in the mineral is a very effective treatment.

Foods Rich in Magnesium – include nuts and seeds (especially squash and pumpkin seeds), dark green and leafy vegetables like kale, chard and spinach, tuna and mackerel, lentils and beans, bananas, avocados and yogurt (make sure the yogurt is of the non-fat or low-fat variety).

For supplements, it is better to take the advice of your physician. Just to give you a pointer, magnesium oxide is the most commonly prescribed oral supplement and daily doses for adults vary between 270 mg and 350 mg.

It would be important to note here that excessive magnesium in your body can also be dangerous and, therefore, it is imperative that you check with your physician for the right dose and form of magnesium oral supplement to take for RLS treatment.

Therefore, magnesium and iron supplements have the potential to prevent cramping and twitching. Magnesium has also been proven to reduce sleep-restricting periodic limb movements (PMLS).

Other Foods Good for Reducing RLS Symptoms

Water - Drinking plenty of water is essential to remain hydrated and, sometimes, just one glass of water can help to relieve RLS symptoms almost instantaneously. Coconut water is even better because not only does it prevent dehydration but also provides electrolytes and some amount of sugar giving your muscles instant energy.

Omega-3 Fish Oils – The fatty acids supplied by Omega-3 fish oils help in the maintenance of healthy cell membranes resulting in a healthy circulatory system. Moreover, omega-3 fatty acids are known to be beneficial to many other organ and organ systems of our body including the immune system, the cardiovascular system, reproductive system and more.

Omega-3 fatty acids are proven through research studies to help balance and heal frayed nerves resulting from prolonged inflammation and protects nerve cells from further complications. Its anti-inflammatory properties help in healing the inflammation that causes RLS symptoms.

Co-enzyme Q10 – This element helps to improve the uptake of oxygen resulting in an improved production of energy in muscle cells. There are two forms of co-enzyme Q10; the ubiquinol form and the ubiquinone form. The former is known to treat RLS symptoms better than the latter one.

Garlic Tablets – Specifically good for the treatment of poor blood circulation, garlic tablets effectively increase the flow of blood through small and narrow blood capillaries and vessels. Garlic contains multiple compounds that help in relaxing the blood vessels and dilating small arteries in a much better way than many other compounds. This increased dilation improves blood flow to peripherals such as nail tips and nail folds.

B Vitamins – B Vitamins are vital nutrients for processing energy in cells. Therefore, it is imperative that you consume foods rich in these B vitamins as part of your daily diet. Multivitamin supplements help to safeguard your body from the negative impacts of micronutrient deficiencies.

B Vitamins are collectively found in yeast extracts, seafood, whole grains, pulses, meat, eggs and more. Let us look at each of the B Vitamins and see which of the foods are rich in each type of Vitamin B:

- *Vitamin B1 (or thiamin)* – Duck and pork are rich in this B vitamin
- *Vitamin B2 (riboflavin)* - Carton milk is a good source of riboflavin. However, excessive exposure to light destroys it.
- *Vitamin B3* – Eggs are a great source of Vitamin B3
- *Vitamin B5 (pantothenic acid)* - royal jelly is rich in this vitamin
- *Vitamin B6 (pyridoxine)* – Bananas, soy products, avocado and walnuts are rich sources of Vitamin B6
- *Vitamin B12* – is found in plenty in kidney, liver, sardines and red meats. Vegetarians are usually prone to the risk of Vitamin B12 deficiency as the only plant source is fortified breakfast cereals and blue-green algae.

Folate, Vitamin B12, and RLS

Low levels or deficiencies of Vitamin B12 and folate are connected to diabetic neuropathy, which is a condition that can trigger RLS symptoms. Research studies have proven that folate and Vitamin B12 supplements along with iron supplements could reduce RLS symptoms and help in its treatment as well. Risk of folate and vitamin B12 deficiency is increased due to malabsorption issues. However, it is also proven that folate deficiencies are rare conditions and are usually associated with iron deficiency.

Folate is found in multiple foods and the following are rich sources of this mineral:

- Spinach,
- Asparagus
- Brussels' sprouts

There are folic acid-fortified food items such as cereals, bread, pasta, flours, and many other grains. Clams and beef liver are known to be the best sources of Vitamin B12. Egg, dairy products and Vitamin B12-fortified cereals are also good sources.

Connection between Obesity and RLS

There are studies, which reveal the connection between RLS and obesity. Studies conducted with participants who did not have diabetes or arthritis (and not pregnant too) revealed that obese people ran a much higher risk of being diagnosed with RLS than those who were not obese.

The connection between obesity and RLS could be the fact that obese people are also prone to increased risk to diabetes, cardiovascular problems and compromised production and release of dopamine. These conditions are all connected to Restless Legs Syndrome. So, it is important that you manage your weight if you want to be relieved or at least reduce symptoms of RLS.

Foods to Avoid

Foods containing caffeine and alcohol should definitely be avoided if you are suffering from RLS symptoms. These aggravate and stimulate nerves and enhance the agony of Restless Legs Syndrome. So, the following foods must be avoided: coffee, tea, chocolate, energy drinks and all forms of alcohol. It is also important to limit intake of the following foods: fried items, soda, high-sugar foods and processed foods.

Other Lifestyle Changes for RLS

Caffeine and alcohol increase RLS symptoms considerably. Avoid these two beverages.

Restful sleep is an essential part of your lifestyle to help to relieve symptoms of RLS. If you overly tire yourself out during the day, severe symptoms of RLS will prevent you from getting a restful sleep

The efficient functioning of your digestive tract is directly connected to RLS. Poor gut flora can trigger RLS symptoms which is the reason why you must avoid processed and junk foods of all kinds. Avoid foods that are connected with bloating, gas, etc.

Find the right kind and the right combination of aerobics and stretches for yourself. Too little exercise and too much exercise are both detrimental to the health of RLS-afflicted people

Stretching your legs before going to sleep can help relieve symptoms of restless legs syndrome

Hot and/or cold packs might help too. Try and experiment with various combinations and use those, which work for you. A warm bath before bedtime may also work.

Quit smoking completely

Massage the affected area (there is another chapter in this book about the various ways you can self-massage).

Sometimes, taking your mind off of the symptoms plaguing you can also be effective. Try a hobby that you enjoy like solving a crossword puzzle or reading, etc

Drugs That Could Trigger RLS Symptoms

There are some drugs that are known to trigger RLS symptoms. It makes a lot of sense to tell your physician about all other drugs that you take but especially if you have been prescribed the following drugs:

- Drugs to prevent nausea
- Antipsychotic drugs
- Antihistamines with sedating effects
- Antidepressants
- Calcium-channel blockers

Summarily, the best chance you have to keep RLS symptoms at bay is to ensure you lead a healthy lifestyle that comprises nutritious food and moderate-to-mild regular exercises.

<u>Here is a small list of do's and don'ts as a reminder:</u>

- Do consume a lot of fresh fruit and vegetables which extra emphasis on leafy dark green vegetables
- Do consume foods rich in iron or take iron supplements after consulting with your doctor
- Do eat legumes, nuts, and seeds daily
- Limit or better still completely avoid processed foods of all kinds
- Don't drink beverages with high levels of sugar or corn syrup
- Don't consume fried foods and other foods that could result in weight gain

Chapter Four:

Herbal Remedies for RLS

There are a lot of herbs and herbal remedies that have known to help in the treatment of Restless Legs Syndrome. They help alleviate symptoms and also are known to cure the medical condition itself, sometimes. It is important to remember that herbal remedies do not work magic overnight and will take time. It is therefore imperative that you persist in your efforts and be patient until the positive effects are felt.

Astralagus

The Astralagus herb belongs to the legume family and has a long proven history of being an immunity booster. It has been used in Chinese medicine for thousands of years to fight off as well as to prevent the onset of various disease conditions. It is a perennial flowering plant and is native to the eastern and northern regions of China. It can also be traced back to Korea and Mongolia.

The Astralagus herb in an ancient Chinese herbal medicine that has been in use for a long time to facilitate increased absorption of iron from digested food. The Astralagus herb is also proven to help improve blood circulation in the body. Also referred to as 'milkvetch,' the Astralagus herb has been used by the Chinese as a general health tonic because of its ability to enhance the functioning of the immune system.

The primary factor of Astralagus herb to be used to treat Restless Legs Syndrome is its amazing ability to increase absorption of iron by the body from the digested food. As a large percentage of patients afflicted with RLS are known to be iron-deficient too, this is a perfect herbal therapy for the condition.

Its other properties include:

- Anti-inflammatory
- Improved Immune System
- Prevents and slows down the growth of tumors
- Protects and improves the functioning of the cardiovascular system
- Regulates and also prevents diabetic conditions
- Is a great anti-oxidant
- Reduces scarring and helps in healing wounds

Butcher's Broom

Named after the fact that its dried leaves were used as brooms across the European Continent, Butcher's Broom's scientific name is Ruscus aculeatus and belongs to the lily species. With properties that are very similar to the asparagus plant, the roots and stems of Butcher's Broom are used to make supplements.

This herb is a native of Iran, the Mediterranean region, some parts of Africa and the Azores Islands. There are some cultures that eat the prepared shoots (just like asparagus) even though the flavor is bitterer than that of asparagus. Other names of Butcher's Broom are pettigree, box holly, knee holly, sweet broom and Jew's myrtle.

This herb is one of the primary treatment for RLS and other blood circulation related disorders in homeopathy. Butcher's Broom works to improve the viscosity of blood thereby improving circulation. It has also been used as a laxative and diuretic.

'Ruscogenin,' a phytochemical present in Butcher's Broom has the potential inhibit 'elastin' resulting in better stability for blood vessels. In addition to being used for RLS, Butcher's Broom is used to treat and relieve the symptoms of hemorrhoids, swollen legs and varicose veins. The primary reason for the effectiveness of Butcher's Broom in the treatment of RLS is because of its anti-inflammatory properties.

An important element to remember about Butcher's Broom is that it can interact with stimulant and blood pressure medication. So, it makes sense to talk to your physician before taking this as part of your RLS therapy.

American Skullcap

The University of Maryland Medical Center recommends the use of American Skullcap in the treatment of RLS because it has been in use for over 200 years as a relaxant. Also known as 'Mad Dog,' this herb is available as teas, tinctures and herbal supplements. It is advised for all kinds of sleep-related discomforts including restless legs syndrome.

American Skullcap has a relaxing and calming effect and is great for use during the day to restore balance in your body if you are overworked. This same relaxing effect is the reason why it is great as a way to alleviate RLS symptoms. This herb which has been in use for a long time in Western cultures is also used to improve moods, immune system, sleep and to reduce stress all of which are associated with RLS.

An important point of note is not to confuse this herb with Chinese Skullcap, which is used for many conditions but can affect the cardiac system. American Skullcap for relieving symptoms of RLS can be drunk as a tea (2-3 cups a day) or taken as oral supplements (2 capsules a day). The supplements are all prepared from the fresh parts of the plant.

This antispasmodic herb which can be used as a natural sedative can promote menstruation and, therefore, should be avoided by children, pregnant women, and people afflicted with hormonal disorders.

Horse Chestnut

This is a Native American tree that grows to an average height of 80 feet. It is an important herbal remedy for RLS. The fruit, the bark, and the leaves of this tree are all beneficial. Yet, the seed extracts from this herb are what is used for treating RLS symptoms because it is filled with natural compounds that improve blood flow and overall health of veins.

Just like other herbs, Horse Chestnut can also be used for a variety of medical conditions especially those related to the veins such as hemorrhoids. Horse chestnut has been used for hundreds of years by Native Americans to cure many diseases such as digestive and bladder issues, fever and cramps in the leg. Its ability to cure and control venous insufficiency is the reason horse chestnut is used to treat RLS and has some great benefits in alleviating pain caused by the debilitating disease.

It is essential to take care that you consume only the commercially available extract of Horse Chestnut as the unprocessed and raw seeds, leaves, and fruit of the tree could be toxic. It is totally to be avoided for use in children, pregnant women and people with kidney disorders.

Passion Flower

This herb is great for reducing the burning sensation that is associated with restless legs syndrome. Combining beauty and functionality, the passionflower, which belongs to the Passifloraceae family, improves the production and release of Gamma-aminobutyric acid, a powerful inhibitory neurotransmitter in the brain.

Those parts of the plant that are above the ground are used in various forms to treat different medical conditions. It is a perennial climbing vine and is native to the southeast parts of America. Now, it is grown a lot in Europe as well. The other names for passionflower include apricot vine, maypop, passiflore and passion vine.

Passion Flower not only relaxes the nerves in the affected area but also on the muscles resulting in a highly effective homeopathic medicine for alleviating RLS symptoms. Passionflower induces relaxation and mild sedation and minimizes the frequency and duration of disturbances that get in the way of restful sleep at night.

In addition to being used for the treatment of RLS, passionflower is used for the treatment of high blood pressure, to reduce hot flushes, anxiety and depression. Its ability to improve sleep is one of the main reasons for it to be recommended for RLS.

The best way to consume Passion Flower herb is to drink one cup of its tea an hour before bedtime, which will ensure alleviation of pain and restful, undisturbed sleep at night. Again, pregnant women and people taking antidepressant drugs should NOT consume passionflower.

Valerian Root

A natural sedative and a highly effective sleeping aid, the Valerian root is a commonly used herb for the treatment of RLS. Valerian root does not work at treating the disorder as much as it works at making the symptoms of the medical condition less disruptive than before.

As it aids in restful sleep, the debilitating effects of RLS symptoms are felt to a much lesser degree than otherwise making it worth your while to take this herb if you are suffering from RLS.

This natural sedative is also known to ease the effects of insomnia, nervous restlessness and anxiety all of which are annoying side-effects of restless legs syndrome. It naturally calms anxious and frayed nerves and reduces blood pressure too.

Fava Beans

Many of the research studies on RLS have been able to connect the medical condition to the levels of dopamine in the body although the exact link is yet to be clearly established. Fava Beans are a rich resource of L-Dopa, a unique and singular element responsible for producing and releasing dopamine in the brain. Therefore, Fava Beans are a natural herbal remedy for RLS as well as brain-related conditions such as Parkinson's disease.

Also referred to as brown beans, these fava beans are an amazing variety of herbs considering the fact that they contain a huge amount of nutrition including Vitamin B6, Vitamin K, copper, zinc, magnesium, iron, and more. Additionally, fava beans are a great source of folates, an important nutritional ingredient for RLS.

Despite the absence of the exact connection between RLS and dopamine, medical experts know and agree that the two are linked in some mysterious ways making fava beans an approved herbal remedy for RLS.

Ginkgo Biloba

This is another wonderful herb, which improves dilation of blood vessels resulting in improved blood flow to the legs and, therefore, an effective therapy for RLS. Also referred to as maidenhair, it is an ancient Chinese herbal medicine that has been in use for thousands of years to heal and cure many ailments.

It is an excellent anti-inflammatory and anti-oxidant (because of the presence of terpenoids and flavonoids) element that also has the power to improve platelet formation and boost blood circulation. Today, the extracts are made with the plant's green but dried leaves. Gingko Biloba protects the body and body parts from oxidative stress and mitochondrial damage.

Padma Circosan

This is a blend of multiple Tibetan herbs and has been approved as a drug in Switzerland for the treatment of circulatory disorders. Padma Circosan facilitates improved blood flow to your legs and also helps to reduce the nasty RLS sensations such as heaviness, tingling, tension, crawling sensations, cramps and numbness. This drug contains over 20 ingredients and has been prescribed by many physicians to relieve symptoms of RLS. Again, like most herbal medicines, this too should NOT be taken by pregnant and/or lactating women or children.

In summary, herbal remedies are effective complementary therapies along with conventional pharmacology. However, it is always a wise thing to speak to and get approval from your physician before trying them.

Chapter Five:

Essential Oils for RLS

With no known cure from the traditional pharmaceutical medication shelf, people suffering from Restless Legs Syndrome are always looking out for alternative therapies to try and relieve painful symptoms. This chapter is dedicated to the use of essential oils as an effective pain remedy for restless legs syndrome.

Essential oils have multiple therapeutic properties such as analgesic, antispasmodic, sedative, calming and anti-neuralgic. These properties help to relieve pain and other RLS symptoms effectively. Additionally, essential oils have a warming effect naturally helping in muscle relaxation and, therefore, are excellent for treating spasms, muscle aches and pains.

Peppermint Essential Oil

Powered by cooling, analgesic and antispasmodic properties, peppermint essential oil is excellent therapy for restless legs syndrome. It relieves muscle pains, aches and spasms.

Peppermint Essential Oil as a Massage Rub – Combine the following essential oils:

- Peppermint essential oil – 2 drops
- Rosemary essential oil – 4 drops
- Black Spruce essential oil – 4 drops

- Carrier oil – 4 tsp

Gently massage this combined oil in at the affected area. There is a chapter later on how to give self-massages. You can use the tips from there to massage in the oil.

Peppermint Essential Oil in a Cold Compress – Take 4 drops of peppermint oil and 4 drops of yarrow oil and put them into 2 cups of cold water. Stir well so that everything is blended well. Dip a small cotton cloth into this mixture and wrap the cold wet towel around the affected area of your leg. If you want to use it for the other leg as well, simply double the amount of ingredients for another cloth.

Lavender Essential Oil

This essential oil has antispasmodic and analgesic properties and is excellent for relieving muscle spasms, aches and pains. Lavender essential oil also has a calming effect, which gives you a deeply relaxed and uplifted feeling. Great to counter ills of insomnia as well, lavender essential oil is a wonderful therapy for restless legs syndrome.

Lavender essential oil bath blend for pain relief – Add 4 drops of the wonderfully aromatic lavender oil along with 2 drops of vetiver essential oil to your bath and enjoy a relaxing bath.

Lavender essential oil bath blend to counter insomnia – Add 4 drops of lavender essential oil and 2 drops of sweet orange oil to your warm bath before bedtime. It works wonders for insomnia relief.

Marjoram Essential Oil

Empowered with sedative, analgesic and antispasmodic properties, Marjoram oil is great for muscle pain relief. It is soothing and comforting as well enhancing its therapeutic effect for restless legs syndrome.

Marjoram essential oil blend for a hot bath – Add 4 drops of marjoram essential oil and 2 drops of vetiver essential oil to your hot bath and enjoy a restful sleep at night.

Marjoram essential oil massage blend – Add 4 drops of marjoram essential oil to 2 tsp of carrier oil and gently massage the affected area.

Vetiver Essential Oil

With natural sedative, calming and antispasmodic properties, vetiver essential oil works well and aromatically to manage muscle pain and spasms. It also stimulates blood circulation, which enhances relief from RLS symptoms. Its deeply calming effect is the primary reason for its excellent work against RLS symptoms.

Vetiver essential oil hot bath blend - Add 2 drops of vetiver essential oil along with 4 drops of sandalwood essential oil to your hot bath for pain relief

Vetiver essential oil massage blend – Combine 2 drops of vetiver essential oil with 4 drops each of neroli and linaloe essential oils and use this mixture to massage the affected area.

Lemongrass Essential Oil

It is a natural sedative and analgesic and, therefore, the perfect remedy for restless legs syndrome.

Lemongrass essential oil diffuser blend – Add 2 drops of this oil with 4 drops of lavender essential oil into a diffuser machine and keep it in your bedroom. The wafting smell will help you have a relaxing sleep.

Lemongrass essential oil massage blend – Combine 2 drops of lemongrass essential oil, 4 drops of ginger essential oil, and 4 drops of lavender essential oil to 4 tsp. of a carrier oil of your choice. Blend the mixture well and massage it into the affected area

Roman Chamomile Essential Oil

With a natural calming effect combined with anti-neuralgic, analgesic, and antispasmodic properties, Roman chamomile essential oil is great oil for relieving RLS symptoms.

Roman chamomile essential oil hot bath blend – Have a nice, relaxing, hot bath with 4 drops or Roman chamomile essential oil and 2 drops of sandalwood essential oil in your bath water.

Roman chamomile essential oil massage blend – Make a blend of 4 drops of Roman chamomile essential oil, 4 drops of lavender essential oil, and 4 tsp. of your favorite carrier oil and massage this oil mixture on the affected area gently.

Roman chamomile essential oil as a cold compress blend - Take 4 drops of roman chamomile essential oil into 2 cups of cold water. Stir well so that everything is blended well. Dip a small cotton cloth into this mixture so that the entire mixture is absorbed into the cloth (or towel). Now, wrap the cold, wet towel around the affected area in your leg. If you want it for the other leg, simply double the amount of ingredients for another cloth or towel.

Frankincense Essential Oil

This essential oil has natural sedative and antiseptic properties. With its power to heal and balance, frankincense essential oil is great for relieving RLS symptoms.

Frankincense essential oil bath blend – Add 2 drops of frankincense essential oil and 4 drops of rose geranium essential oil to your bath water and have a relaxing bath.

Frankincense essential oil massage blend – Add 8 drops of frankincense essential oil to 4 tsp of your favorite carrier oil and blend well. Then, massage it gently on the affected area.

Ginger Essential Oil

It is naturally warming oil and is great for stimulating blood flow. Also, powered by antispasmodic, neuralgia and analgesic properties, you can happily use ginger essential oil to help you alleviate symptoms of RLS.

Ginger essential oil massage blend – Combine 2 drops of ginger essential oil, 4 drops of black pepper essential oil, 4 drops of cardamom essential oil, and 4 tsp. of your favorite carrier oil. Massage this oil blend gently on to the affected area.

Ginger essential oil hot bath blend – Add 2 drops of ginger essential oil and 2 drops of lavender essential oil to your hot water bath and enjoy a relaxing bath just before bedtime.

Jasmine Essential Oil

With natural antispasmodic and analgesic properties, jasmine essential oil with a sweet, floral, rich and heady fragrance is a wonderful therapy for RLS symptoms.

Jasmine essential oil hot bath blend – Add 2 drops of jasmine essential oil along with 2 drops of sweet orange essential oil to your hot bath water for good relief from RLS-related pains and agony.

Jasmine essential oil massage blend – Make a massage blend with 6 drops of jasmine essential oil and 4 tsp. of your favorite carrier oil and massage the affected area gently.

Rosemary Essential Oil

With a natural warming tendency along with antispasmodic and analgesic properties, rosemary essential oil is calming as well, making it a great oil to use for RLS symptoms relief.

Rosemary essential oil massage blend – Combine 4 drops of rosemary essential oil, 4 drops of black pepper essential oil, and 2 drops of vetiver essential oil and mix well. Massage this oil mixture on the affected area.

Rosemary essential oil hot bath blend – Add 2 drops of rosemary essential oil and 3 drops of lavender essential oil to your hot bath water.

Black Pepper Essential Oil

Black pepper essential oil is replete with natural antispasmodic and analgesic properties. Along with its natural warming effect, this essential oil is great for RLS symptom relief.

Black pepper essential oil massage blend – Make a massage blend with 2 drops of black pepper essential oil, 4 drops of rosemary essential oil, 4 drops of lavender essential oil and 4 tsp. of carrier oil. Massage this oil mixture gently on the affected area.

Black pepper essential oil diffuser blend – Add 3 drops of black pepper essential oil and 3 drops of mandarin essential oil to a diffuser. Fix the diffuse in the room of your choice and breathe in the therapeutic smells of this combination.

Black pepper essential oil hot bath blend – Add 2 drops of black pepper essential oil and 2 drops of jasmine essential oil into your bathwater before going for your bath.

Basil Essential Oil

Basil essential oil is great to relieve deep muscle pains due to its powerful and natural antispasmodic properties.

Basil essential oil massage blend – Combine 4 drops of basil essential oil, 4 drops of lavender essential oil, 2 drops of black pepper essential oil and 4 tsp. of carrier oil and massage this blend gently on the affected parts of your leg.

Bergamot Essential Oil

With natural calming, analgesic, and antispasmodic properties, bergamot essential oil is great to relieve muscle pains and aches. It is also a wonderful muscle relaxant and, therefore, a good bet to reduce painful RLS symptoms.

Bergamot essential oil massage blend – Make a massage oil by combining 2 drops of bergamot essential oil, 4 drops of jasmine essential oil and 4 drops of sandalwood essential oil and gently massage the affected parts of your leg with it.

Bergamot essential oil hot bath blend – Add 2 drops of bergamot essential oil and 2 drops of neroli essential oil to your bath water for a relaxing bath just before bedtime.

Clove Essential Oil

Clove essential oil has natural anti-neuralgic, analgesic and antispasmodic properties. Powered with the ability to stimulate blood flow, it is an excellent remedy for RLS.

Clove essential oil massage blend – Combine 2 drops of clove essential oil, 2 drops of cinnamon leaf essential oil and 6 drops of bergamot essential oil and massage this oil mixture gently on the affected leg areas.

Yarrow Essential Oil

An anti-inflammatory agent along with being an antispasmodic and an analgesic, yarrow essential oil is great for RLS.

Yarrow essential oil cold or hot compresses – Add 4 drops of yarrow essential oil to 2 cups of either cold or hot water (depending on which compress you want). Stir the mixture so that it is blended well. Dip a small piece of cotton cloth or towel into this mixture so that all of it is absorbed by the cloth. Now, wrap it around the affected area in your leg. Simply double the quantities if you want another hot or cold towel.

Yarrow essential oil massage blend – Combine 6 drops of yarrow essential oil with 4 tsp. of any carrier oil of your choice. Blend well and massage it on the affected leg area.

General Instructions for Using Essential Oils

When using essential oils topically (such as for massaging), you must remember to blend with a carrier oil and not directly massage the essential oil into your skin. Clove and rosemary oils are best avoided by pregnant and lactating women. If you have other health problems including but not limited to epilepsy, hypertension, etc., please speak to your physician before using any of the essential oils mentioned here.

Also, any citrusy essential oil can be very sensitizing to your skin and, therefore, you must be careful while using it. Use such oils in very small amounts. Always run a patch test with all new essential oils before using it to identify any allergic reactions that might occur.

Nature does have her valuable resources to help people afflicted with RLS to alleviate their symptoms and these wonderful essential oils are just a representation of nature's limitless bounties.

Chapter Six:

Yoga for RLS

This chapter is dedicated to giving you some basic yoga poses and exercises that are known to help reduce RLS symptoms. So, let's dive right in.

Legs-Up-the-Wall Pose or the Inverted Lake Pose or Viparita Karani

This pose is great for RLS because it improves blood circulation to every part of your body. This is perfect for people who are sitting or standing the entire day at work and if done in the evening can reduce RLS symptoms and get you a disruption-free restful sleep at night.

Lie on your back. Extend your legs up and lean them at a 90-degree angle against the wall. Extend your arms on the floor as well. Use the wall to ensure support for your upward extending legs. Stay in this position for as long as you can starting from the 2-3 minutes and slowly increasing the duration up to 20 minutes.

Beginner's Tip – Initially, it might be difficult for you to balance on the wall. Here is a tip that will help you in the beginning learning stages. Make sure the top of the thigh bones are pressed firmly on the wall which will act as a great support for the groin, spine and belly areas giving you the necessary balance to keep your inverted legs slanted against the wall.

Pose Variations – If there is sufficient place, then you can make a V with your outstretched legs, which will increase the stretch in the muscles of your thigh and groin area. Another way to increase the stretch in your hamstring muscles is to bend your knees and bring the soles of your feet together. Then, slide the feet down and try to touch the pelvis area with your heels.

Benefits of the Inverted Lake Pose

- It relaxes the cramped and tired legs and feet and, therefore, perfect for RLS
- It can relieve mild backaches too
- It soothes and calms the mind (again great for RLS)

Contraindications - This pose is not allowed for people with high blood pressure, for pregnant women, or if you are in your menstruation cycle.

Standing Forward Fold or Standing Forward Bend or Uttanasana

The primary idea of this asana is to stretch your calf muscles and as this is one of the most affected parts of your body when you have RLS, this asana is perfect for relief. Stand erect with your feet as wide apart as the width of your hips. Now, slowly bend forward at the hips and while keeping your knees straight (not stiff but soft and straight), fold your spine forward and bring your face to come between your ankles.

Use your hands to hold the ankles for support. Hold for 5 breaths initially (or even a lower number if you are not comfortable for this length of time) and slowly increase the duration to hold for up to 10 breaths. Slowly get back to the original position. In fact, coming up again should be done at a very slow speed. Suddenly, reverting your head back to the top might cause giddiness.

Again, this asana should not be tried if you are being treated for high blood pressure.

Beginner's Tip – In the beginning, it might be difficult to bend forward with ease. In the initial days of learning, you can bend your knee slightly to achieve the effect. With practice, you will find it easier to bend down to your ankles while keeping your knees straight.

Pose Variations – These are advanced pose variations and not to be tried until you have mastered the basic pose. This advanced pose will increase the stretch at the back of your legs and you will feel improved relief from RLS symptoms. Lift your body and stand on the balls of your feet as you slowly pull your heels up about half an inch from the floor. Hold this position for a couple of breaths.

Benefits of the Standing Forward Bend

- This asana gives a great stretch to your back, hamstrings, and your calves all of which will directly benefit RLS patients
- It relieves anxiety and calms your mind
- It is a great treatment for insomnia and headaches
- Your knees and thighs will gain in strength

Contraindications – This asana is to be avoided if you have an injury in your lower back, a hamstring tear, sciatica or glaucoma.

Seated Forward Fold or Seated Forward Bend or Paschimottanasana

Again, the calf muscles and your hamstrings are stretched in this asana and, therefore, it is really good for RLS symptoms relief. Sit on the floor or on a yoga mat with your feet extending in front of you. Now, increase the length of your spine by making yourself erect and bend forward at the hip while trying to clasp your hands around your feet.

If you cannot reach forward enough to clasp your hands around your feet, use a towel or belt around your feet and hold the ends of it in your hands. Use your legs and feet to balance and stabilize your body. Focus on stretching your calf, hamstring, and spine and not so much on bending forward.

Beginner's Tip – It is perfectly alright not to be able to get it right the first, second, or even after multiple attempts. As you try to bend forward and you notice that the space between your pubis and your navel is reducing, simply lift yourself a little and continue to move forward. Stiffness in the leg muscles will make it difficult initially. But as you keep practicing, the stiffness will reduce and you will find it easier to bend forward much more with each attempt.

Pose Variations – The clasping of your hands around your feet is actually an advanced pose variation. In the beginning, simply try and touch your toes while you keep your elbows bent. As you become better at this asana, you can straighten your elbows and clasp your hands around your feet. This will call for a lot of bending in the forward direction and, therefore, will take time, effort and lots of practice. However, even with the basic pose mastered, you will find a lot of relief.

Benefits of the Seated Forward Fold

- It's great to treat mild depression as it soothes an anxious and calm mind
- The hamstrings, calves, and the spine get a good stretch.
- Fatigues, headaches, and anxiety are reduced
- This asana is great for women after they have childbirth

Contraindications – If you have a back injury, diarrhea, or asthma, please avoid this asana. Pregnant women are not advised not to try it.

Seated Forward Fold Variation or Janu Sirsasana

You must start this pose the same way you started the seated forward bend asana. However, in this asana, bend one knee (we'll start with the left leg bent) and hold the left leg beside the right leg and keep only the right leg stretched out in front of you.

You can use a blanket to support the folded leg. Now, lengthen your spine, inhale deeply, and bend forward at your hip so that you try and touch the toes of your right leg with your hands. Hold this position for about 5-10 counts before getting back to the original position slowly and gently. Now repeat with your left leg too.

Beginner's Tip – Always make sure the foot of your bent leg is touching the straight leg. It should not be under that leg lest it adds undue pressure to the other leg. When you bend forward and look down, you must be able to see the sole of your leg that is bent.

Make sure your bent leg doesn't go to sleep while you are focusing on the straight leg. The heel of this leg should touch the inner groin area of your straight leg and you must focus on this touch to ensure the bent leg is active.

Pose Variations – To increase the stretch, you should look at increasing the angle formed between your straight leg and the bent leg. Slowly increase the angle until you reach 90-degrees.

Benefits of the Seated Forward Fold Variation

- The shoulders, the hamstrings, and the groin area are stretched well
- Digestion improves a lot because all the digestive organs are massaged well with this asana
- It helps counter effects of insomnia and anxiety

Contraindications – If you have asthma or diarrhea or a knee or back injury or a lumbar disc herniation, it is not advised to do this asana.

Supported Bridge Pose or Setu Bandhanasana

Lie flat on your back and bend your knees. Your feet should be flat on the ground and as apart from each other as the width of your hip. You can use a pillow to support your lower back. Now, lift your back off the ground as high as you can. Use your hands, which are on either side of you as a lever to push yourself up at the hip. Hold this position for 5-10 counts.

Beginner's Tip – When you try to roll your shoulders in order to lift your body up, remember the shoulders must not be pulled away from the ears in a forceful manner. This can result in overstretching the neck and cause discomfort at that region. Gently lift your shoulders toward your ears even as you try and push the shoulder blades away from your spine. This will give you the lift needed to get your hip off the ground.

Pose Variations – When you are comfortable with the basic pose, then you can lift one foot off the ground and hold it outstretched above your head. Repeat with the other leg.

Benefits of Setu Bandhanasana

- It stretches the muscles of your back and releases the knots and kinks there.
- It reduces anxiety, stress, and depressive moods
- It improves blood circulation

Contraindications – People with a neck injury, pregnant women (a toned down version is allowed but only under the supervision of a trained practitioner) and people with back problems must not do this asana.

Child's Pose or Balasana

Kneel on the floor. Sit on your heels. Keep your arms folded at the back or you can keep them resting at your side. From this position, straighten your torso and move it forward and bend at your hips to try and touch your forehead to the floor. If you cannot bend forward so much, keep rolled blankets at the place where your forehead will touch the floor.

Rest in this position for a couple of minutes initially and as you gain comfort and master the pose, you can rest like this for up to 20 minutes. You must have noticed that many babies sleep like this for hours. That is what is being replicated in this asana.

Beginner's Tip – This asana will help you learn to breathe fully through your torso and stomach. This asana is a great one to practice to get ready for the other more difficult forward bend poses.

Pose Variations – Instead of having your hands at the back or beside you, you can stretch and straighten them over your head and place them on the floor with your palms touching the ground.

Benefits of Balasana

- It stretches the muscles of the shoulders, chest, and back
- It reduces anxiety and stress
- It stretches and lengthens the spine
- It relieves pain in the neck and in your back
- It promotes blood circulation

Contraindications – If you have knee injury or are suffering from diarrhea or are being treated for high blood pressure, then this asana is not for you.

Basic Relaxation Pose or Shavasana

Lie on your back on a blanket or your yoga mat. Keep rolled blankets under your knee and/or your arms for extra support. Your hands must be outstretched and lying on the sides with the palms facing upward. Ensure your head is comfortably positioned on the floor or mat. Close your eyes, breathe gently, and relax every part of your body starting from your toes and moving up to your head. You can stay in this position for as long as you want because this pose is meant for only relaxation, especially after every yoga session.

Beginner's Tip – There is nothing much to tell here except to give in to the deep relaxation allowed by this asana. Breathe normally without stress and enjoy the relaxed feeling

Pose Variations – If you feel uncomfortable because your head might be slightly lower than your neck (especially if you are using a bolster), then you can raise the head to the same level by using a pillow or a rolled blanket. This will help in relaxing the neck muscles.

Benefits of Shavasana

- It brings your entire body into a deeply meditative state which is ideal for RLS
- It is a wonderful way to end your yoga workout
- It reduces anxiety and blood pressure
- It boosts energy
- Yoga poses and postures create a lot of information that go back and forth between the nervous and the muscular system of our body. The Shavasana pose is the perfect time for the body to integrate the messages and information to help balance all the systems in our body.

And finally, finish your yoga session with some deep breathing exercises that will improve the state of calmness in your mind.

Contraindications – This asana is absolutely safe and everyone and anyone can practice it. Pregnant women should use a bolster or cushion for the neck and chest.

Chapter Seven:

Self-Massages for RLS

Massage is a very useful and valuable tool to alleviate RLS symptoms. The most difficult symptom of RLS is the overwhelming desire to move your legs. If you manage to move your legs, the effect removes the stress for a little while. Many people tend to walk around in the night while others move or stretch their legs. Massage is another option too and this chapter is dedicated to giving you some tips on how to self-massage so that you feel better.

The Effectiveness of Massaging for RLS

Treatment and relief measures for Restless Legs Syndrome is quite nuclear as the reasons or causes for the condition are also not yet known. While some experts believe that a lowered level of dopamine is a big contributor, some others people that lifestyle, genetic conditions, etc. could be contributory factors as well and these affect the severity and frequency of RLS symptoms.

Also, it is clear that moving the affected limb does provide some amount of relief. Some particular types of movements provide faster relief than other kinds of movement. In fact, some kinds of movement do not do anything to relieve pain and uncomfortable sensations. For example, when the desire to move the leg is overwhelming, some patients feel relief when they move, but the sensations and discomfort come back as soon as the effect of moving the leg stops.

Research has proven that temperature and tactile stimulation help a lot to relieve RLS symptoms and also help the patients from being disturbed during sleep. Massages are perfect to achieve these two effects of temperature and tactile stimulations. Here are some of the advantages of massages and how they help in relieving RLS symptoms:

- After the massage is completed, dopamine is released into the bloodstream thereby helping in relieving RLS discomforts
- Massages are also proven to stimulate the cerebral cortex which is another reason why it might be beneficial for RLS-afflicted people
- Massaging is also known to activate the functioning and efficacy of the thalamus. As this important organ is believed to play a crucial role in the frequency and severity of RLS, massages are an effective therapy for RLS.
- Sometimes, it is possible that the act of gentle massages might achieve the stimulation needed by the nerves and muscles in the affected area.
- Massages are very relaxing. Since both anxiety and stress seem to be contributory factors for RLS, the relaxing effect of massages help in reducing symptoms

Basic Movements to Use in Your Self-Massages

- At the beginning and end of the massage session, use *effleurage* or long and sweeping strokes on the affected area
- When you have to work your muscles, use **petrissage** or muscle rolling and kneading movements like kneading dough.

- When you have to reach deep inside through layers of skin and fat, use *friction* which is applying deep pressure at one particular point using knuckles, thumbs or fingertips
- *Tapotement* or rhythmic tapping or percussion-like movements help in increasing the muscle stimulation in the area

All these basic massage movements can be used when you self-massage the affected areas for RLS symptoms relief.

Areas to Self-Massage and Techniques

Calf Muscles – The calf area in both your legs are the best places to start your self-massage. There are different methods to massage the calf muscles. You can use a roller or a hard ball to move your muscles over it so that any kinks in the area can be removed. You can also simply massage the calf muscles with your fingers and remove any kinks and knots you feel. Make sure every part of the calf muscle is massaged including the sides.

Hamstring Muscles – Hamstrings are also known to a play a role in Restless Legs Syndrome. Therefore, massaging the hamstring muscles is a good way to work out kinks there, which will relieve RLS symptoms. Massaging of the hamstring muscles is done with fingers usually. However, you can use rollers or a ball to smoothen out the knots. If you are massaging with your fingers, remember to go deep into the skin layer because, at the hamstrings, there is a lot of fat and thick skin before you can reach the muscles.

Heated Massages – The effect of integrating massages with heat is better than doing only the massage. After all, RLS symptoms can be reduced by stimulation of temperature and tactility. Remember not keep the hot towel very hot lest it burns your skin. Keep the towel moist. Additionally, if you are already being treated for other medical conditions such as diabetes, heart disease or high blood pressure, then you must first speak to your physician before you apply heated massages.

Stone Massages – Another way of self-massaging is to roll a hot stone over the affected area. You can heat up the stone either in a crock-pot or in a skillet that is at least 3 inches thick. You must take extreme care when you are doing stone massages as hot stones can scald your skin. If you are not comfortable, avoid doing this. Moreover, it might make sense to go to a professional and get a good massage for yourself regularly, especially if you are affected by RLS.

In summary, self-massaging is the easiest and cheapest way to stimulate the relevant parts of the affected areas and other parts of your body so that you can get some relief from the painful symptoms of RLS. Self-massaging for RLS has another benefit. You can feel the effect of the massage as you do it and make appropriate changes immediately.

If some strokes are working well, you can increase them and if some strokes are painful or are not very effective, you can stop using them. Whether proven to be efficacious or not, it is important to remember that during a painful RLS episode, self-massages are great to try and feel the relief from agony and pain, at least for the period you are doing it.

Chapter Eight:

Other Home Remedies for RLS

Although there are no conventional cures for Restless Legs Syndrome, you must now be convinced that there are many lifestyle, nutritional, exercise and natural elements like essential oils that can reduce the painful impact of this rather debilitating disorder. Here are some more natural remedies for RLS that you can try at home.

Change Your Diet

In addition to following the nutritional advice and suggestions given in an earlier chapter of this book, look closely at what you are eating and drinking. Identify ingredients and food elements that could trigger symptoms. Study your diet and find out what you are sensitive too. Moreover, if you are already being treated for another medical condition such as diabetes, hypertension, etc. but they are not being managed properly, then the symptoms of RLS will worsen.

So, it is imperative that you look at your diet really, really closely and ensure you remove all elements that are not good for you. Stick to healthy, home-cooked meals as much as possible. Excessive sugars, salts, oil, refined flours, etc. must be completely avoided.

Include a lot of iron-rich and magnesium-rich foods like beans, collard greens, kale, avocados, spinach, peas, dried fruit, seafood, poultry and red meat. Include a lot of Vitamin C-rich foods such as citrus fruits, melons, strawberries, broccoli, rice, quinoa, tomatoes and peppers in your daily diet. Vitamin C helps in better absorption of iron.

If you look at the foods that are mentioned above, you will notice that a good combination of some or all of the ingredients will give you balanced and healthy meals with the right mixture of macro- and micronutrients needed for your body. A healthy diet is anyway a great way to improve overall health, which, in turn, will improve other ailments, and disorders that are troubling you and/or aggravating RLS symptoms.

Do Not Miss Out on Your Exercise

Follow the instructions and tips given in this book and ensure you get your exercise regimen right every day. Working out and exercising releases endorphins or happy chemicals, which, in turn, improve dopamine levels in the body resulting in, reduced RLS symptoms. Sedentary poses such as sitting or lying down for a long time trigger RLS discomfort and exercises help in countering this.

Whether it is in the form of stretches and aerobic exercises or in the form of yoga or anything else that suits you, do not miss out on your daily exercise regimen. It is also important to do your exercises earlier in the day because sweating it our close to bedtime can actually enhance RLS symptoms.

Take Your Mind off RLS

RLS is known to create and/or enhance anxiety levels in people. Thoughts such as "I hope I am able to sleep well without being disrupted by aches and pains," or "I hope I can sit through the entire movie without getting cramps," plays on your mind so much so that your mind is completely preoccupied with your medical condition, sometimes even when there is no need.

To counter this, it is important to take your mind off RLS and get distracted. There are research studies that prove the efficacy of mental games and puzzles to help you to get distracted. Find mentally stimulating games such as reading, crossword puzzles, computer work, card games, knitting, or even have meaningful conversations with people you like, so that your mind is focused on something other than RLS-related anxious and stressful thoughts.

Leverage the Power of Mindfulness

There are many mindfulness based stress-reducing techniques (MBSR) that are known to help RLS-affected patients handle their symptoms in a better way than before. Experts teach patients how to manage stress-creating symptoms before they take place. Being mentally prepared for the symptoms helps many patients. For example, MBSR techniques teach patients to tell themselves, "Yes, I know that the symptoms will come. But I'm going to accept them and do my best to try and reduce them by working with them instead of against them." These mindfulness techniques have helped people get improved and less disrupted sleep than before.

Identify Medicines Playing Havoc

Check your medicines and see which drugs could cause RLS triggers. There are many drugs that are known to play havoc in RLS patients. So please check your medicine cupboard/box and remove all those drugs. Some of the drugs that have the potential to trigger RLS symptoms include anti-emetics (to fight nausea), antidepressants, antihistamines and antipsychotics.

When you approach your physician for help with Restless Legs Syndrome, please make sure you tell him (or her) whatever medications you are taking including the alternative medicines and over-the-counter drugs. Follow your physician's orders strictly when it comes to medication.

While most of the generic drugs mentioned here are bad for RLS, it is possible that your physician might have an alternative medicine for these disorders that don't aggravate RLS symptoms.

Avoid Alcohol and All Other Stimulants

Nicotine, alcohol and caffeine are all stimulants that exacerbate RLS symptoms. There are multiple studies that prove that people who don't drink or smoke are prone to lesser pain and discomfort from RLS symptoms. Many experts opine that giving up alcohol, nicotine and caffeine altogether can help in managing RLS symptoms much better than otherwise.

High-Tech Gadgets

Thanks to advanced technology, there are a few gadgets (approved by the regulatory authorities) that help to reduce RLS symptoms. These non-drug treatment options are electronic pads. The pads emit timed vibrations that are designed to counter and balance the body's stimulation. Of course, studies have yet to be conducted to record and observe the efficacy of these pads.

Probiotics

There is a very strong connection between gut health and RLS even though the exact nature of the link is yet to be established. Probiotics such as live-culture kefir and yogurt increase the good and healthy flora in the gut, which helps in increased absorption of nutrients from the digested food. These beneficial gut flora also help to fight against the disease-causing microbes and bacteria.

People who are afflicted with celiac diseases are known to be at a higher risk of getting RLS. Therefore, intolerance to food items such as gluten, lactose, etc. can be countered using probiotics in addition to avoiding consumption of the ingredients as well.

Iron and Magnesium

I have already spoken of the connection between iron, magnesium and RLS. Yet, it might make sense to include it here as well because both these elements seem to be directly responsible for RLS and ensuring you get the right amounts in your system will keep the disorder and its negative impacts at bay. It is essential that you take supplements only after consulting with your physician. Do NOT self-medicate.

Hot and Cold Compression

There have been many reports from patients regarding hot/cold compressions combined with hot baths before bedtime as being helpful in managing RLS symptoms. Adding essential oils, baking salts, Epsom salt, sea salt, etc. to your hot bath before bedtime can be an effective measure to counter uncomfortable RLS symptoms.

Practice Proper Sleep Hygiene

RLS symptoms make it very difficult to have an undisturbed restful sleep. Ensure that you don't make it worse by being undisciplined about your sleep habits. Fix a regular time to go to bed. Make sufficient time to do your pre-bedtime rituals including a hot bath, self-massages, etc. Slow down mentally and physically well before your bedtime. Stop using your electronic devices about an hour before you go to sleep.

Make a good bedtime ritual like listening to soft music or reading which can lull you to sleep. You need to focus your energies to identify what works best for you. Use various trial and error methods and find one that suits you best and stick to it diligently. Look at your bedroom and eliminate all sleep-disturbing elements from it including TV, cell phones, alarm clocks, etc.

More Sleep Tips

- Sleep at a regular time so that your body and mind get the hint when it's time to sleep
- Try and use a pillow between your legs while sleeping. This might give some support to the nerves and muscles in that area thereby helping in the reduction of RLS symptoms
- Try and change your mattress. You can use natural latex or memory foam, which is great for relieving pressure points in your body as you lie down. These mattresses have another advantage. Your partner will not be disturbed by your movements, which could be frequent considering the nasty effect of RLS.
- Try and change your blanket too. A heavy blanket might actually help at calming the nerves in your legs. The heaviness of the blanket gives you a sense of 'hugging' comfort that could help reduce painful symptoms

Meditation

Any chronic stress has the ability to increase the risk of RLS as well as making the symptoms worse than before. The reason for this could be that stress hormones keep muscles constantly in a state of tension. Deep breathing exercises and meditation help calm muscles and nerves thereby facilitating the reduction of RLS symptoms. Allocate some regular time every day for meditating and find a quiet, peaceful place to do it. You will see a huge improvement in your sense of calmness after a few regular meditation sessions.

Things to Avoid for RLS

Caffeine, alcohol and nicotine should be avoided as much as possible, preferably completely

Avoid overdoing exercises. High-impact and high-intensity exercises should NOT be done. In the same vein, it is important to reduce exercising slowly if you have been big on exercise before being diagnosed with RLS. For example, if you have been walking three miles every day, don't suddenly stop altogether. Reduce your miles slowly and taper them to something that is more doable.

Avoid taking medications without your doctor's prescription and advice.

Conclusion

Yes, there are a lot of approved medications that do reduce the pain and discomfort for the duration of their effect. When the effect wears off, you will have to take the medication again. It makes sense to try and combine the medications with natural home remedies so that your dependency on chemicals that cause a lot of negative side effects is reduced.

The side effects of these medicines include weight gain, dry mouth, brain fog, fatigue and more all of which are as nasty as the symptoms of Restless Legs Syndrome. Moreover, there is evidence that after a couple of years or so, these medicines cease to be effective. Of course, newer pain medications are constantly being researched and invented. Yet, none of them are without nasty side effects.

And as you age, the symptoms are only going to get worse and countering them with medication alone will not really help. It is always good to find alternative methods to reduce symptoms of RLS, which could be complemented with conventional medications occasionally.

If you are undergoing a lot of pain because of RLS, it might just be that you are suffering needlessly because of lack of knowledge to combat the pain or keep it at bay. This book, I hope, will open your eyes to a lot of alternative, cheap and fairly beneficial remedies that you can try at home itself.

Remember that any disease, especially chronic ones, can make your life miserable for you only if you allow it. If you steel your mind and take steps to fight against it, you will find your iron will is capable of coming to your rescue more often than not. So, go on and take that step to fight back.

Bonus!

Free e-Book!

Would you like a bonus gift? As a "Thank you" for getting this book I would like to offer you an e-book for free, as a gift. Just follow the link below and you will immediately get your free bonus e-book *"10 Tips for Healthy and Happy Feet"*. Enjoy reading!

Follow The Link Below and Download Your Free e-Book:

http://eepurl.com/dufnan

Resources

https://www.healthline.com/health/restless-leg-syndrome/treatments

https://www.webmd.com/brain/restless-legs-syndrome/restless-legs-syndrome-rls#2

http://www.naturallivingideas.com/12-natural-remedies-restless-leg-syndrome/

https://www.sitandbefit.org/exercises-restless-leg-syndrome/

https://www.everydayhealth.com/sleep-disorders/restless-leg-syndrome/10-ways-exercise-with-restless-legs-syndrome/

https://drsarahbrewer.com/health/restless-leg-syndrome-remedies   https://www.healthline.com/health/restless-leg-syndrome-diet#lifestyle-changes

https://www.healthline.com/health/restless-leg-syndrome/link-between-magnesium-and-rls

https://www.everydayhealth.com/hs/rls-management/healthy-diet-for-restless-legs-syndrome/

http://nourishholisticnutrition.com/coping-with-restless-leg-syndrome/

https://www.herbs-for-health.com/herbs-for-restless-legs/

https://www.up-nature.com/blogs/news/17-powerful-essential-oils-for-restless-leg-syndrome

https://www.everydayhealth.com/sleep-pictures/yoga-poses-for-restless-legs-syndrome.aspx

https://www.findatopdoc.com/Healthy-Living/Relaxation-Techniques-to-Alleviate-Restless-Legs-Syndrome

http://www.stylecraze.com/articles/balasana-child-pose/

http://www.progressivehealth.com/rls-massage.htm

https://www.prevention.com/health/home-remedies-for-restless-leg-syndrome

https://www.thesleepjudge.com/sleep-tips-bedding-guide-rls/